The
Matcha
MIRACLE

Boost Energy, Focus and Health
with Green Tea Powder

The
Matcha
MIRACLE

Boost Energy, Focus and Health with Green Tea Powder

DR. MARIZA SNYDER, DR. LAUREN CLUM AND ANNA V. ZULAICA

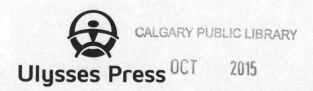

Ulysses Press

Published in the US by:
Ulysses Press
P.O. Box 3440
Berkeley, CA 94703
www.ulyssespress.com

ISBN13: 978-1-61243-486-5
Library of Congress Control Number: 2015937559

Printed in Canada by Marquis Book Printing
10 9 8 7 6 5 4 3 2 1

Acquisitions editor: Kelly Reed
Managing editor: Claire Chun
Editor: Renee Rutledge
Proofreader: Lauren Harrison
Cover design: Rebecca Lown
Interior design: what!design @ whatweb.com
Cover artwork: green and white border © miumiu/shutterstock.com, green tea
    © joephotostudio/shutterstock.com
Layout: Lindsay Tamura

Distributed by Publishers Group West

NOTE TO READERS: This book has been written and published strictly for informational and educational purposes only. It is not intended to serve as medical advice or to be any form of medical treatment. You should always consult with your physician before altering or changing any aspect of your medical treatment. Do not stop or change any prescription medications without the guidance and advice of your physician. Any use of the information in this book is made on the reader's good judgment and is the reader's sole responsibility. This book is not intended to diagnose or treat any medical condition and is not a substitute for a physician.

Contents

• •

Introduction

Alert calm. Together, the two words seem to form an oxymoron. In American culture, alertness is associated with paying close attention, being ready to act, and inhabiting a state of vigilance, whereas calm is associated with ease, peace, and quietude. While the two are not mutually exclusive, they're not often tied together. However, being able to achieve an alert calm state can bring about considerable productivity and innovation. This concept of alert calm is exactly what makes matcha green tea powder so unique.

Matcha green tea powder is literally ground up green tea leaves. It has been used for centuries to create a tea beverage in which the entire (ground) tea leaf is dissolved in hot water, as opposed to traditional tea drinks where tea leaves are soaked in hot water. While the latter method will inevitably reap significant nutritional goodness from the tea leaves into the beverage, the former offers tenfold the nutritional benefit by mixing the entirety of the tea leaf directly into the drink.

The traditional preparation of a tea beverage is still the most popular use of matcha green tea powder and is a phenomenal way to experience the rich taste and astounding health benefits of this special tea. However, innovation abounds in our culture and people have become more and more creative with the powder, expanding its uses into a variety of sweet and savory recipes for beverages and foods. Popular blogs, magazines, and food companies have featured matcha green tea powder in lattes, smoothies, pastries, and even cocktails! As you flip through this book and our recipes, you'll find distinctly healthy dishes incorporating this special powder.

In addition to offering an abundance of healthy recipes, the goal of this book is to give a thorough understanding of matcha green tea powder. Matcha's history and evolution are explained, along with common uses over the course of time, and perhaps its most compelling characteristic, the amazing health benefits it presents.

Clinical practice has shown us time and again that while recipes look and sound delicious, and can spur creativity and new ideas, it's understanding the background of a healthy food that truly motivates one to incorporate it into daily routines. In fact, it was matcha's background that truly inspired us to write this book! As it has gained popularity and clients have begun asking us about it, we were forced to study it beyond our general understanding that it was high in antioxidants. And as we began researching, we ourselves became more and more motivated to add it into our own daily rituals! We hope the same will be true for you—that you will be inspired by matcha's ease of use and amazing health benefits, as well as the creative recipes that this book presents.

CHAPTER 1

History of Matcha Tea

During the Song Dynasty in China (960–1279), powdered tea was developed and became popular. Little pieces broken off of bricks of tea called "tea cakes" were whisked into hot water to create drinking tea. The tea cakes were made by first steaming fresh tea leaves, which preserved their color and freshness. A mud or paste was formed by drying the steamed leaves and grinding them into a powder, and molded into a cake by being left in the sun to harden, and then baked. Tea cakes were not only easy to make, but easy to transport and store.

Zen monks from Japan traveled through China during this time and were introduced to the powdered teas. They started bringing the tea cakes, along with seeds for tea plants, back to Japan, in order to utilize and grow tea at home. It wasn't long before Zen priests began their own tea traditions, developing systems and processes for cultivating and preparing powdered tea.

One Zen priest in particular, Eisai, is credited for initiating the cultivation of matcha tea in Japan in the 11th century. Over the course of time, matcha became Japan's most treasured type of green tea, reserving its role as the only tea to be used in the traditional Japanese tea ceremony.

This traditional Japanese tea ceremony, termed *Sadō*, or "the way of tea," was popularized due to use within Samurai society, royalty, and the upper class of Japan. It was developed by Zen monks over the course of the 15th century, and is based in large part on four guiding principles: harmony, purity, tranquility, and respect. While other types of green teas are grown throughout the world, matcha green tea powder is cultivated only in Japan, utilizing traditional farming, sourcing, and grinding methods. During the final few weeks of springtime harvesting, the tea plants are covered by bamboo mats to limit their exposure to sunlight. The decreased sunlight increases the plants' chlorophyll content, contributing to the dark green color of the leaves and vibrant spring green of the final matcha green tea powder. While increasing the plants' potency, covering them also weakens them, meaning that they need more time to recover before being harvested again.

Japan is a small country to begin with, offering only so much land on which to grow tea leaves, and they only export 1 percent of their teas because of high domestic demand. As such, traditional matcha green tea powder tends to be more expensive than other green teas and green tea products.

Tea Grades

Once the matcha tea plants have been harvested, the leaves are steamed then air-dried. The leaves then get sorted, with the smaller, softer, younger top leaves going toward premium matcha powder and the larger, firmer, more robust bottom leaves slated for ingredient-grade matcha. The stems are removed and the leaves deveined, producing tencha, which is the precursor to matcha. While most tencha leaves are ground into matcha, some of the harvested leaves are made into green tea. Tencha is a unique green tea: it is harvested from the first flush of a tea plant that has been kept shaded, and is steamed, but not rolled. (The most common type of green tea, sencha, is steamed and rolled soon after harvesting.)

The highest-quality matcha is ground with a stone mill, producing a fine powder consisting of uniquely shaped granules. Stone-ground matcha is typically used for making tea, as the consistency of the powder impacts the final taste and feel of the tea beverage. Machines can be used to grind the tea leaves as well, producing what is called industrial-grade or ingredient-grade matcha. While this matcha powder may be suitable for use in cooking and baking recipes, it's going to have a distinctly different taste and feel in your tea.

	Tea-Grade	Industrial- or Ingredient-Grade
Made From	Young, small, soft, top leaves	Firm, robust, bottom leaves
Consistency	Very fine, unique granules	Not as fine, consistent granules
Best Uses	Making tea to drink	Baking and cooking recipes
Where to Find	Online, Asian markets	Grocery store
Expense	More expensive	Less expensive

Tea grade matcha is typically divided into two categories: thin and thick. While at first it seems that these descriptions would just denote texture of the liquid, they actually describe the character and style of the tea. *Usucha* is thin matcha, and is prepared with more water (2 to 3 ounces) and less tea (1.5 chashaku scoops, or ½ teaspoon), and may or may not produce a frothy head. *Koicha* is thick matcha, is prepared with less water (1½ ounces) and more tea (3 chashaku scoops, or 1 teaspoon). It requires a slower, stirring motion and does not produce the foamy froth that usucha does. Koicha is typically made with more expensive matcha from older tea trees and produces a milder, sweeter flavor than usucha. It is used almost exclusively in traditional Japanese tea ceremonies.

Preparation

To this day, matcha green tea powder is highlighted in traditional Japanese tea ceremonies, or Sadō. The custom of preparing and serving matcha green tea, both for the ceremony and just in general in Japan, is very different from just pouring some hot water over a tea bag—the common tea preparation in the US. The following outline for preparing matcha green tea stems from the Sadō ritual and is a good guideline for maintaining the integrity of the powder. Storing, preparing, and serving traditional matcha green tea begins with the appropriate equipment. The powder should be stored in an airtight, lighttight container in the refrigerator. The traditional tea caddy is called *natsume*. Traditional utensils include the *chawan*, a ceramic tea bowl, the *chasen*, a bamboo whisk, and the *chashaku*, a tea scoop. A tea sifter is also sometimes used, in case the powder is at all clumpy.

First, hot water is added to the chawan to heat it up. After a few minutes, the water can be discarded and the tea bowl dried with a *chakin*, or special tea cloth. One to two scoops of matcha green tea powder is then added to the chawan with the chashaku, followed by 1 to 3 ounces of hot (not boiling) water, depending on whether you're making thin or thick tea. The mixture is then briskly whisked with the chasen until a frothy head forms at the top of the tea. At this point, it is ready to drink and should be tasted with a hearty slurp.

The taste of matcha is described as grassy, spinachy, and/or vegetal, and produces what's called the fifth taste, *umami*. Translated from Japanese, umami means "pleasant savory taste" and is described as an agreeable brothy or meaty flavor with a long-lasting, mouth-watering coating sensation over the tongue.

CHAPTER 2

Matcha Green Tea Benefits

• •

Matcha has been a time-honored "health elixir" for over 900 years in Japan and is renowned for numerous health benefits, many of which have been researched extensively. The secret behind matcha's super strength and incredible benefits are found in the high concentration of antioxidants contained in one cup of matcha tea. According to the latest research on antioxidants, matcha green tea is 10 times more nutrient-dense than regular green tea, and the health benefits make it one of the most potent superfoods in the world. In understanding the role of matcha for the body, it's important to understand exactly why antioxidants, as a whole, are critical to optimal cellular vitality, how they can play a major role in health, and why adding this simple daily habit into your life through the easy, delicious recipes found in this book is so important.

Antioxidants come up frequently in discussions about good health, antiaging, and disease prevention. These powerful vitamins, polyphenols, and enzymes are mostly produced from plant-based sources such as raw fresh fruits, vegetables, and herbs. Antioxidants consumed on a daily basis prohibit and prevent the oxidation of other molecules in the body, known as free radicals. The benefits of antioxidants are very important to good health because if free radicals are left unchallenged and unneutralized, they can cause a wide range of degenerative illnesses and chronic diseases.

Free radicals are the by-products that our bodies create naturally as they process the food we consume. Additional free radicals develop when we're exposed to environmental toxins, such as pesticides, radiation pollutants, synthetics, and ultraviolet rays. Even stress can produce additional free radicals in the body. Although antioxidants created in the body are designed to counteract free radical damage, all too often the number of free radicals, produced naturally or from environmental stressors, far outnumber the naturally occurring antioxidants that the body produces. In order to maintain a healthy balance of antioxidants to free radicals and obtain the maximum benefits of antioxidants, a continual supply of external sources of antioxidants is necessary.

Antioxidants increase energy, slow the aging process, lead to younger-looking skin, and prevent a number of life-threatening chronic diseases. Our first book, *The Antioxidant Counter*, studied the benefits of antioxidants and provided an in-depth reference guide to the ORAC (Oxygen Radical Absorbance Capacity) scale. The ORAC scale measures the concentration of antioxidants in many common foods and beverages.

Amazingly, just one cup of matcha green tea provides over five times as many antioxidants as any other food. In fact, it's the highest-rated food by the ORAC scale. Experts at Tufts University discovered that matcha scores up to 1,573 units on the ORAC scale. Matcha green tea possesses antioxidant levels 6.2 times that of goji berries, 7 times that of dark chocolate, 17 times that of blueberries, and 60.5 times that of spinach!

• •

ORAC Scores of Top Antioxidant Foods in ORAC Units per Gram

(ORAC = Oxygen Radical Absorbing Capacity)

Matcha: 1,573

Goji berries: 253

Dark chocolate: 227

Wild blueberries: 93

Spinach: 12.6

• •

Matcha tea leaves store an abundance of natural antioxidants and polyphenols. A research study assessing the antioxidant power of matcha green tea reveals that as compared to other green teas, matcha has the highest amount of epigallocatechin gallate (EGCG), an extremely powerful antioxidant with significant health benefits. EGCG is a specific type of catechin found in superfoods like green tea, cocoa, and blackberries. Heralded for being more catechin-dense than most items, green tea (and especially matcha) provides unbelievable health benefits for people who regularly drink it. In the world of antioxidants, EGCG is more potent than either vitamins C or E individually, and actually assists the vitamins in doing their jobs. The catechins and polyphenols present in matcha are 100 times more potent than in vitamin C and 25 times more potent than in vitamin E, according to research out of the University of Kansas.

Matcha green tea is a high-nutrient food. Aside from catechins, matcha also contains vitamin A, vitamin B-complex, vitamin C, vitamin E, vitamin K, trace minerals, other polyphenols, and chlorophyll. It also contains amino acids L-theanine and theophylline. The nutrient properties in matcha have been linked to a myriad of benefits for the body. These benefits range from improved energy and sleep quality to protection against infections and improved cardiovascular health. We are going to explore each important benefit so that you can gain clarity on just what matcha can do for you with occasional to daily consumption. The recipes in chapter 4 (page 19) will not only taste great, but pack a nutrient punch.

Since catechin is the "secret" super-antioxidant ingredient found in matcha tea leaves, let's dig further into the research that exists today. Researchers at the National Cancer Institute (NCI) discovered that catechins in matcha green tea (EGCG, EGC, ECG, and EC) may actually help prevent cancer. In their extensive research, the NCI provides the following explanation:

1. The constituents in green tea, especially EGCG and ECG, have substantial free radical scavenging capability and have been proven clinically to protect cells from DNA damage caused by reactive oxygen species.

2. Tea polyphenols have also been shown to inhibit tumor cell development and induce apoptosis (cancer cell destruction) in laboratory and animal studies.

3. The catechins in green tea activate detoxification enzymes, such as the glutathione and S-transferase family, and quinone reductase, which are praised for preventing tumor growth.

4. Research has supported that the catechins in green tea not only protect against damage caused by ultraviolet (UVB) radiation, but can also improve immune system function.

Immune System Support

Matcha green tea contains incredible immune-boosting properties in every cup. Like many antioxidants, catechins in the form of EGCG have a multitude of healing properties on a cellular level. These same EGCG catechins are also effective in fighting against various bacterial, viral, and fungal infections. Specific investigative research suggests that EGCG binds to the lipid membrane and exerts inhibitory action against growth of various important human pathogens, including influenza A virus, hepatitis B and C viruses, herpes virus, adenovirus, *Staphylococcus aureus* bacteria, and *Candida albicans* yeast. EGCG catechins have also been linked to boosting immune function with specific nutrients. Just one cup of matcha green tea provides substantial quantities of potassium, vitamins A and C, iron, calcium, and enzymes. Further studies have even suggested that EGCG catechins in matcha may have the ability to inhibit the attack of HIV on human T cells. In the same research, it is noted that consumption of matcha green tea may also help in protecting the brains of HIV patients. This protection is attributed to the penetration power of EGCG through the blood-brain barriers, a feat which is not feasible for synthetic and commercially available antiretroviral drugs.

Healthy Heart and Blood Glucose Levels

Matcha green tea may prove valuable for maintaining heart health, metabolism, and blood sugar levels in individuals with diabetes and cardiovascular conditions. The EGCGs in matcha green tea have been shown to aid in reducing the levels of triglycerides, total cholesterol, and hepatic glucose content in individuals with diabetes. In studies looking at different populations, it's been demonstrated that people who drink matcha green tea on a regular basis have lower levels of LDL (bad) cholesterol while at the same time displaying higher levels of HDL (good) cholesterol. A 2011 study featured in the *American Journal of Clinical Nutrition* demonstrated that administration of green tea beverages or extracts significantly lowered serum total cholesterol (lowered total cholesterol levels in the serum and liver, along with LDL cholesterol and LDL). A newer study shows men who drink matcha green tea are 11 percent less likely to develop heart disease than those who don't.

Perfectly Balanced Energy Booster

Matcha green tea provides a well-balanced energy boost for your morning ritual. For centuries, matcha green tea has been used to create a sense of alertness while the body feels calm and relaxed, enhancing energy without caffeine jitters. It contains a healthy form of caffeine not to be mistaken with the one present in regular coffee. This unique form of caffeine, known as theine, is derived from the tea plant *Camellia sinensis*. Half a teaspoon of matcha contains approximately 35 milligrams of caffeine, which is significantly less than coffee, which contains 80 to 150 milligrams. Due to its unique combination of phytonutrients, the caffeine in matcha is assimilated in a very different and much healthier way than caffeine from coffee. The caffeine in matcha binds to its larger catechin molecules and is released into the bloodstream slowly over time as the catechins are broken down and assimilated. This slow release supports the functionality of adrenal glands and maintains optimum hormonal levels in individuals, impacting cortisol in particular. The result produces a sustained energy for three to four hours. This mechanism also prevents insulin and cortisol spikes typical of coffee intake, so the "crash" that occurs when blood sugar levels drop simply does not happen.

Weight Loss

When it comes to boosting metabolism and helping with weight loss, few things are more beneficial than matcha green tea's high concentration of catechins. A 1999 study featured in the *American Journal of Clinical Nutrition* demonstrates that green tea extract rich in catechins has thermogenic properties and promotes fat oxidation beyond that explained by the tea's caffeine content. This study found that consuming matcha green tea can increase thermogenesis (the body's unique rate of burning calories) from a typical 8 to 10 percent of daily energy expenditure to between 35 to 43 percent of daily energy expenditure. Another study demonstrates that exercising immediately after drinking matcha green tea results in 25 percent more fat burning during exercise.

Detoxification

An important reason to drink matcha green tea every day is to promote detoxification. The precious matcha tea plants are shaded from direct sunlight for two to four weeks before harvest. The result is a substantial increase in chlorophyll content within the leaves of the matcha plant. Chlorophyll is an excellent cleanser to detoxify cells in the body. It aids in maintaining the alkalinity of blood and tissues. Chlorophyll also helps in preventing the integration of harmful toxins within colon walls and flushes those toxins out of the body. Matcha naturally removes heavy metals and chemical toxins from the body through the specific nutrients it contains.

Memory and Concentration Boost

For over a millennium, matcha green tea has been used by Japanese Zen Buddhist monks as a means to relax and meditate while remaining alert. Now we know that this higher state of consciousness is due to the amino acid L-theanine. L-theanine is a unique amino acid found almost exclusively in the matcha green tea plant and is the primary amino acid component of green tea. The shading of the tea plants before harvest increases the L-theanine content, giving matcha its characteristically lovely and sweet flavor. L-theanine promotes the production of alpha waves in the brain, which induces relaxation by inhibiting neuron excitation, producing a relaxed physiological state. Clinical studies have also shown L-theanine can reduce stress levels, lower blood pressure, improve memory and focus, diminish PMS symptoms, and promote beneficial antioxidant activity in the brain. Another side effect of L-theanine is increasing the natural production of dopamine and serotonin. These two neurotransmitters serve to enhance mood, improve memory, and promote better concentration.

CHAPTER 3

Using Matcha

Traditional teas are made by steeping tea leaves in hot water. Nutritional benefits occur as the leaves impart their goodness to the water. Matcha green tea leaves are ground up in a stone mill to produce a fine powder that actually dissolves in hot water when a cup of tea is made. By consuming the entirety of the leaves dissolved into the very water that you're drinking, you increase the nutritional bounty tenfold. You read that right—you'd have to drink 10 cups of traditional green tea to approach the nutritional benefit of just one cup of tea made with matcha green tea powder!

While matcha green tea powder is currently the most popular type of tea powder, consuming teas made from powders is not a new concept. Matcha green tea was originally introduced by China to Japan at the end of the 1100s. Long before that, as early as the 7th century, the Tang Dynasty in China made tea from a powder that was formed from tea leaves that were steamed, formed into bricks, roasted, then pulverized. Three hundred years later, the Song Dynasty, also in China, popularized the tea-making method of whipping hot water with the tea powder, very similar to what is done today. Preparing and consuming powdered tea was ritualized by Zen Buddhists who are responsible for bringing the methodology, along with matcha green tea, from China to Japan in 1191.

As you've learned, the abundance of antioxidants in matcha green tea is a big part of what makes this potent powder so very healthy. However, antioxidants are not indestructible, and if their delicate structure isn't taken into consideration during food preparation, their potency can take a major decline. While matcha green tea powder is a phenomenally healthy ingredient, it doesn't automatically impart its health properties to whatever it's mixed into. Variables such as cooking temperatures, cooking times, and other ingredients must be taken into consideration in order to honor and maintain the veritable health of the green tea powder.

In a general study of a variety of antioxidants in 20 different types of cooked vegetables, it was found that some antioxidants, such as vitamin C, decrease with any amount and any type of cooking, whereas others, such as lycopene and carotenoids, increase with moderate temperatures. Another study looked at several different groupings of antioxidants specifically found in red peppers and how the cooking methods of stir-frying, roasting, steaming, and boiling impact antioxidant levels. The study concludes that all cooking methods decrease the values of all of the types of antioxidants, some more than others. The most offensive cooking method is boiling, which destroys the highest number and type of antioxidants. The least offensive cooking method is stir-frying, which preserves the majority of most of the types of antioxidants. Overall, it appears that cooking vegetables on the stovetop, on a griddle, or in a pan at a medium temperature for a short period of time produces the least amount of destruction to the vegetables' antioxidant content. On the flip side, boiling vegetables for a long period of time creates the most destruction of antioxidants across the board.

Now, how the heck do we relate those somewhat confusing findings to matcha green tea powder? The reality is that there haven't been studies specifically analyzing the impact of temperature and cooking times on the powder, so we have to deduce that the similar antioxidant properties in matcha green tea powder would react similarly to those in vegetables when put into similar circumstances. As such, we've crafted our recipes to preserve as much antioxidant and nutritional power as possible by minimizing cooking temperatures and times. Flipping through our recipes, you'll find lots of raw recipes, where no cooking is needed at all! For those recipes that inevitably require cooking, we've attempted to minimize the temperatures and cooking times in order to preserve the green tea powder's antioxidant content.

Another variable that can affect or impede matcha green tea powder's nutritional power punch is the use of other ingredients. Some ingredients are so egregious, so devoid of nutrition that including them completely negates the health benefits of the powder. A great example is buttercream frosting. The sheer amount of sugar in such a recipe makes it an unhealthy option; it doesn't matter how much matcha green tea powder or any other wildly healthy ingredient you add to that much sugar—it is never going to be a healthy recipe! As such, you will not find recipes in this book that use ridiculously large amounts of unhealthy ingredients, such as refined white sugar and refined white flour. We've gone out of our way to devise scrumptious dessert recipes for you that not only preserve the nutritional value of the matcha green tea powder, but incorporate other healthy ingredients and minimize the devastatingly unhealthy options.

Regardless of what health claims a particular food can make, whether accurate or not, it must fit into a larger scheme of health reasoning in order to be utilized at its full potential. Again, it would be silly to suggest that any dish can be made healthy by simply adding matcha green tea powder! That's just not how health and healing work!

You'll find that all of our recipes fall in line with our food philosophy, which includes a few simple rules. Eat real, whole food, or foods made from real, whole food. Eat an abundance of plants in a variety of colors and an abundance of healthy, brain-building, heart-supporting fats.

CHAPTER 4

Recipes

Our collection of delicious recipes includes a mixture of healthy cooking trends, such as Paleo-friendly, vegan, gluten-free, and more. Please note that not all of the recipes are all of these things! The recipes fall on a scale of being very simple to a bit more complicated. None are overly complicated, and all have been tested by average people, not just chefs! Just by being open-minded enough to incorporate matcha into more and more everyday dishes, you are already setting yourself up to be a better chef, a smarter, more aware consumer, and most importantly, a healthier person.

A Note About Ingredients

Not all matcha green tea powders are created equal! Matcha meant for drinking will be very fine, not clumpy or in need of straining. Less expensive options are available and are reasonable choices if it's being added to recipes rather than made into tea. If you find that all you have on hand is ingredient-grade matcha (page 4), you can still make tea! Just push the powder through a fine-mesh strainer before adding water.

We recommend that most if not all of your ingredients be organic and pesticide free. Locally grown fruits and vegetables that are in season are also preferred. It is true that some produce absorbs toxins and pesticides more than others, so seek out a trusted guide of which conventional produce is reasonable compared to which should always be bought organic. Herbs are on the "always organic" list, as their delicateness makes them more susceptible to pesticide absorption. Buying locally and seasonally reduces your carbon footprint, helps support local farms and growers, and ensures the most nutrition out of the produce.

Eggs: When at all possible, eggs should be organic and from pastured chickens. If you have a highly sensitive soy allergy, check with your farmer to see if the chicken feed contains soy. Oftentimes, pastured eggs purchased at a farmer's market are the most cost-effective option for eggs. Choose cage-free eggs from a reputable source if pastured eggs are not an option.

Oils and fats: All oils used should be organic and cold-pressed. This combination ensures maximum nutrient availability and absorption. Extra virgin olive oil should be used for low-heat cooking or as a finishing oil. Olive oil that smokes when overheated has turned into trans-fat and should be discarded. For high-heat cooking, use extra virgin, cold-pressed coconut oil, high-quality clarified butter (ghee), or organic, grass-fed butter. As long as you utilize the oils or fats noted in a given recipe, you will be using the best option.

Sweeteners: Raw honey is recommended as a sweetener in many recipes. Honey is a superfood that has antiviral and antibacterial properties. Utilizing raw, local honey has been shown to help those suffering with seasonal allergies. If you are pregnant or have a compromised immune system, talk to a doctor before using unpasteurized honey in raw preparations. If raw honey is not an option, maple syrup or coconut palm sugar are great alternatives that are nutrient-dense and more easily assimilated by the body than table sugar. Do not substitute refined white sugar for the sweeteners suggested in the recipes.

Salt: Sea salt contains a wide variety of natural minerals and vitamins that come from the ocean. The more color the sea salt grains contain, the more nutrients they have. Do not be afraid of using sea salt in recipes! It is different from table salt and is good for you, rather than harmful, as many people are told. If sea salt is not available or an option, kosher salt is a good alternative.

TEA

• • • • •

Matcha green tea powder is a very traditional beverage in Asian cultures and it has become more abundant, available, and popular globally. To start, you will find a classic matcha green tea recipe, serving as the foundation to your matcha green tea creations. Rather than sticking to the classic though, also included are creative teas inspired by other cultures, spices, and even textures that you are sure to enjoy.

Classic Matcha Tea
• •
MAKES 2 (8-OUNCE) SERVINGS

16 ounces filtered water

1 teaspoon matcha green
tea powder

raw honey, to sweeten
(optional)

Heat the water in a small pot over medium heat; do not boil.
Meanwhile, place ½ teaspoon of matcha green tea powder into
each of the 2 teacups. Add 2 ounces of the hot water to each cup
and whisk until frothy. Add the remaining water to each cup and stir.
Add honey if desired.

Ginger-Lemongrass-Mint Matcha Tea

● ●
MAKES 2 (8-OUNCE) SERVINGS

16 ounces filtered water

2-inch piece of ginger, peeled and thinly sliced

1 lemongrass stalk, outer leaves peeled off, dark green ends cut off, and white ends cut into 1-inch pieces

6 to 7 mint sprigs, including stems, roughly torn apart

1 teaspoon matcha green tea powder

raw honey, to sweeten (optional)

Heat water, ginger, lemongrass, and mint together over medium heat; do not boil. As the water is about to boil, turn off the heat and let the mixture steep for 3 to 4 minutes. Meanwhile, place ½ teaspoon of matcha powder into each of the 2 teacups. Remove the ginger, lemongrass, and mint from the water. Add 2 ounces of hot water to each cup and whisk until frothy. Add the remaining water to each cup and stir. Add honey if desired.

● ● ● ● ● ● ●
TIP: *For more concentrated flavor, steep the ginger, lemongrass, and mint for longer, and/or do not remove them from the water when adding the matcha powder.*

Matcha Chai Tea

•••••••••••••••••••••

MAKES 2 (8- TO 12-OUNCE) SERVINGS

16 ounces filtered water

2 cinnamon sticks

½-inch piece of ginger, peeled and cut into ⅛-inch-thick slices

seeds from 4 large green cardamom pods

4 whole cloves

3 star anise

¼ teaspoon black peppercorns

1 teaspoon matcha green tea powder

raw honey, to sweeten (optional)

½ cup milk (optional)

Heat water, cinnamon, and ginger in a small pot over medium heat. Then, in a small sauté pan over medium-high heat, add the cardamom seeds, cloves, star anise, and black peppercorns. Toast the spices, shaking the pan every 10 seconds, until fragrant, then add to the pot of water. As the water is about to boil, turn off the heat, stir in the milk, if using, and let the mixture steep for 3 to 4 minutes.

Meanwhile, place ½ teaspoon of matcha powder into each of the 2 teacups. Remove cinnamon, ginger, cardamom seeds, cloves, star anise, and black peppercorns from the hot water. Add 2 ounces of hot water to each cup and whisk until frothy. Add the remaining water to each cup and stir. Add honey if desired.

••••••

TIP: *This recipe works with any type of milk! And for more concentrated flavor, steep spices for longer, and/or do not remove them from the water when adding the matcha powder.*

Iced Vanilla Almond Milk Latte

MAKES 2 (8-OUNCE) SERVINGS

2 ounces filtered water

1 teaspoon matcha green tea powder

raw honey, to sweeten (optional)

1 cup ice

14 ounces vanilla almond milk (see recipe for Homemade Matcha Nut Milk on page 32)

Heat water in a small pot over medium heat, removing the pot from the heat just before boiling begins. Place ½ teaspoon of matcha powder into each of the 2 teacups. Add 2 ounces of hot water to each cup and whisk until frothy. Add honey at this point if desired (the heat will help to dissolve the honey). Then add ice to each cup and pour milk over the ice. Enjoy immediately.

TIP: *The Homemade Matcha Nut Milk can be replaced with any other type of milk.*

SMOOTHIES AND ADULT BEVERAGES
• •

Using frozen produce instead of ice will offer a more flavor-concentrated smoothie. Oftentimes, frozen fruits and veggies can be purchased in bulk at a cost savings, or large quantities can be purchased at the farmer's market and frozen to avoid spoilage and prolong the availability of ingredients.

Superfood Smoothie

• •

MAKES 2 (16-OUNCE) SERVINGS

1½ cups unsweetened almond milk

4 large kale leaves, stems removed and torn into small pieces; or 1 cup baby kale leaves

1 small banana, peeled

½ cup fresh blueberries or strawberries

1 tablespoon chia seeds

1 teaspoon maca powder

2 teaspoons matcha green tea powder

¼ teaspoon ground cinnamon

¾ to 1 cup ice

Combine the milk and kale in a blender and blend on high speed until the kale is broken down. Add the remaining ingredients and blend until smooth. Divide into 2 glasses and enjoy immediately.

Matcha Green Machine

MAKES 2 (16-OUNCE) SERVINGS

16 ounces filtered water, divided

1 cup spinach

3 kale leaves, stems removed and torn into small pieces

½ large avocado

1 small banana, peeled

10 mint leaves

1½ teaspoons matcha green tea powder

½ teaspoon spirulina powder

½ cup ice

honey or 2 to 3 dates (pits removed), to sweeten (optional)

Combine 1 cup of water, spinach, and kale in a blender and blend on high speed until smooth. Add remaining water and other ingredients and blend until smooth. Divide into 2 large glasses. Can be stored in the refrigerator for up to 24 hours.

Antioxidant Powerhouse

● ●

MAKES 2 (16-OUNCE) SERVINGS

16 ounces filtered water

4 large kale leaves, stems removed and torn into small pieces

½ cup acai berry juice

1 cup mixed berries, frozen or fresh

2 teaspoons matcha green tea powder

1 teaspoon cold-pressed organic coconut oil

¾ cup ice, if using fresh fruit (optional)

Combine the water and kale in a blender and blend on high speed until the greens are broken down and smooth. Then add the remaining ingredients and blend until smooth. Divide into 2 large glasses and enjoy within 24 hours. Store in the refrigerator if not consuming immediately.

Probiotic Matcha Shot

MAKES 2 (3-OUNCE) SERVINGS

6 ounces cold goat or cow's milk kefir

2 teaspoons matcha green tea powder

In a small bowl, combine the ingredients and whisk until the green tea powder is incorporated. Divide into 2 small glasses and enjoy immediately.

TIP: *Drink on an empty stomach for maximum absorption of probiotics from the kefir.*

Homemade Matcha Nut Milk

MAKES 3 TO 4 CUPS

1 cup raw, unsalted almonds, cashews, and/or Brazil nuts

4 cups filtered water, plus more for soaking nuts

1 tablespoon matcha green tea powder

½ teaspoon vanilla extract

½ teaspoon ground cinnamon

Place nuts in a small bowl and add filtered water until they're just covered. Place the bowl in the refrigerator and soak the nuts overnight or for at least 4 hours. The nuts will soften and plump up. Larger nuts will need to soak longer.

After soaking, discard water and add nuts to the blender. Add 4 cups of filtered water and the matcha powder, vanilla, and cinnamon. Blend on low for 30 to 45 seconds or until smooth. The nut milk is now ready and can remain unstrained and stored in the refrigerator in a glass container. It should be stirred before drinking.

For an even smoother nut milk, cover the mouth of a large glass container with a cheesecloth, nut milk bag, or fine-mesh strainer and pour the mixture from the blender in batches into the container, straining and using a spatula to push the contents through as needed. Reserve the pulp to dehydrate and use in other recipes, or discard.

TIPS: *Soaking nuts is very beneficial for gut health! Soaking promotes enzymatic reactions in the nuts that begin a sprouting phase, which increases their nutritive potential and removes phytic acid, allowing for better absorption of the nutrients in the nuts. Use almonds, cashews, or Brazil nuts—be creative!*

Chocolate Matcha Shake

· ·

MAKES 2 (10-OUNCE) SERVINGS

16 ounces canned coconut milk

1½ tablespoons unsweetened cocoa powder

1 tablespoon matcha green tea power

2 tablespoons raw honey

1½ cups ice

2 teaspoons cocoa nibs, for garnish (optional)

Combine all ingredients in a blender and blend on high until smooth. Pour into 2 large glasses and top each with 1 teaspoon of cocoa nibs, if using. Enjoy immediately.

· · · · · · ·

TIP: *Cocoa nibs not only provide a beautiful garnish, but a satisfying crunch and antioxidant boost.*

Matcha Piña Colada

MAKES 2 (10-OUNCE) SERVINGS

8 ounces canned coconut milk

4 ounces coconut water

1 cup pineapple

1 tablespoon matcha green tea powder

1 cup ice

2 tablespoons raw honey, to sweeten

2 ounces white rum (optional)

Combine all ingredients in a blender and blend on high until smooth. Divide into 2 large glasses and enjoy immediately.

Honeydew Mint Cooler

MAKES 2 (16-OUNCE) SERVINGS

12 ounces filtered water

1 cup honeydew, cut into
½-inch pieces

10 to 14 mint leaves

2 tablespoons lime juice

2 tablespoons raw honey

1 tablespoon matcha
green tea powder

½ cup ice cubes

2 ounces rum or vodka
(optional)

Combine all the ingredients in a blender and blend on high until smooth. Divide into 2 large glasses and enjoy immediately.

TIP: *You can substitute any melon or other fruit for the honeydew. Choose what you love or what's in season!*

Cucumber Basil Cooler

• •

MAKES 2 (16-OUNCE) SERVINGS

12 ounces filtered water

1 cup English cucumber, peeled and cut into ½-inch pieces

4 to 6 Italian basil leaves

2 tablespoons lime juice

2 tablespoons raw honey

1 tablespoon matcha green tea powder

½ cup ice cubes

2 ounces vodka (optional)

Combine all the ingredients in a blender and blend on high until smooth. Divide into 2 large glasses and enjoy immediately. For a smoother beverage, strain this blended mixture before drinking.

BREAKFAST

• • • • • • • • • • • • •

We always hear "Breakfast is the most important meal of the day." Not only does this first meal kick-start your metabolism and provide you with the energy for the day, but it is also a great opportunity to choose wisely what you eat and it's a chance to pack your body full of vitamins and minerals. In the following recipes, matcha green tea powder is utilized in a variety of sweet and savory dishes that will make the most simple or advanced cook or baker very pleased with the end result.

Matcha Chia Pudding

MAKES 1 SERVING

⅛ cup chia seeds

¾ cup almond milk

½ banana, sliced into half moons

1 teaspoon shredded, unsweetened coconut

1 teaspoon sliced, raw almonds

½ teaspoon matcha green tea powder

½ teaspoon ground cinnamon

In a small bowl, combine all of the ingredients, mixing well. Refrigerate mixture for at least 30 minutes, or until the chia seeds turn into a gel-like substance and look creamy. Mix again and enjoy. Pudding can be left in the refrigerator overnight and enjoyed the next morning. Just mix well before serving.

TIP: *Add more almond milk if you prefer thinner pudding. Or, if you enjoy thicker pudding, consider mashing your bananas!*

Green Yogurt and Superfood Bowl

MAKES 2 SERVINGS

2 tablespoons dried goji berries

1½ cups whole milk Greek yogurt

1 teaspoon matcha green tea powder

1 teaspoon maca powder

½ cup fresh blueberries

¼ cup fresh raspberries

2 tablespoons raw chopped Brazil nuts

Rehydrate the goji berries by placing them in a small bowl and covering with hot water. Allow to soak for at least 10 minutes, or until they are softened. In a separate bowl, combine the Greek yogurt with the matcha and maca powders until fully blended. Drain the goji berries and discard the water, then add them to the yogurt along with the remaining ingredients. Divide into 2 bowls and enjoy immediately.

TIP: *If you want to make this at night for breakfast the next morning, just leave the chopped nuts out of the mixture and add them in the morning!*

Breakfast Toast

· · · · · · · · · · · · · · · · · ·

MAKES 2 SERVINGS

2 slices sprouted whole-
grain bread

½ cup ricotta cheese

1 teaspoon matcha green
tea powder

2 tablespoons raw honey

pinch of sea salt

Toast bread to desired crispiness, either in a toaster or a preheated
350°F oven for 3 to 5 minutes. Spread half the ricotta cheese onto
each piece of toast, then drizzle each with 1 tablespoon of honey,
sprinkle each with ½ teaspoon matcha green tea powder and sea
salt. Enjoy immediately.

· · · · · ·

TIP: *Alternatively, mix the ricotta cheese with the matcha green tea
powder, honey, and sea salt, then divide the mixture between the two
pieces of toast.*

Breakfast Power Balls

● ●

MAKES ABOUT 15 (1½-INCH) BALLS

¼ cup goji berries

3 cups dates, pitted

¼ cup raw Brazil nuts

¼ cup shredded
unsweetened coconut

2 tablespoons coconut oil

3 tablespoons chia seeds

1 teaspoon maca powder

4 teaspoons matcha green
tea powder, divided

4 to 5 tablespoons
unsweetened coconut
flakes, for rolling

pinch of sea salt

Rehydrate the goji berries by placing them in a small bowl and covering with hot water until soft, about 10 minutes. Drain the water, but don't squeeze the berries dry. Add rehydrated goji berries, pitted dates, Brazil nuts, shredded coconut, coconut oil, chia seeds, maca powder, 2 teaspoons of the matcha powder, and pinch of sea salt to a food processor and pulse, pushing down mixture as needed until it is mostly smooth and looks like a paste.

Combine remaining the matcha powder with the coconut flakes in a shallow plate. Wet your hands slightly and make small balls from the paste by pinching off a small amount and rolling it between your palms. Roll each ball in the matcha/coconut mixture and place on a cookie sheet. Enjoy immediately, or store covered in refrigerator for up to 1 week, or covered in the freezer for up to 2 weeks.

● ● ● ● ● ●

TIPS: *Those with allergies can substitute the Brazil nuts in this recipe with any raw nut or seed, or even cocoa nibs. Also, consider chopping the dates by hand before adding them to a food processor if it's not a powerful one.*

Poached Eggs on Matcha Vegetable Hash

MAKES 4 SERVINGS

For the hash:

2 tablespoons ghee

2 large sweet potatoes (about 1 pound total), cut into ½-inch cubes

1 large red bell pepper, diced

1 large yellow bell pepper, diced

½ large yellow onion, chopped

1 bunch dinosaur kale, stems removed and cut into ¼-inch-thick ribbons

3 large garlic cloves, minced

⅛ teaspoon chile pepper flakes

½ cup vegetable broth

1 tablespoon red wine vinegar

1 teaspoon matcha green tea powder

1 teaspoon sea salt

cracked black pepper, to taste

For the poached eggs:

filtered water

1 tablespoon white vinegar

pinch of sea salt

4 large eggs

1 tablespoon Matcha Chimichurri (page 60) (optional)

To make the hash:

Add ghee to a large skillet over medium heat. Once the ghee is hot, add the sweet potatoes and sauté for about 6 to 8 minutes, or until browned on all sides. Add the bell peppers and onion and sauté 3 to 4 minutes, or until browned. Add the kale, garlic, chile pepper flakes, broth, and vinegar, then cover with a lid for 3 to 4 minutes. Remove lid and continue to cook, allowing liquid to evaporate. Add the matcha powder, salt, and pepper, then turn off the heat and cover to keep warm.

To make the poached eggs:

Fill a small pot one-third full of water. Add vinegar and salt and heat until bubbles start to form. Lower the heat so that water is on the brink of a rolling boil. Using a small slotted spoon, swirl the water in a circular motion, then crack an egg right into the center of the swirling water. (To avoid splashing, crack the egg into a ramekin first then pour it into the center of the swirling water.) Allow the egg to cook for 3 to 4 minutes, then lift the egg out of the water with the slotted spoon. Repeat with the rest of the eggs, storing cooked eggs on a paper towel–lined plate to soak up excess water.

To plate:

Place one-quarter of the hash onto each of the 4 plates, top with a poached egg, then spoon the Matcha Chimichurri on top if using. Enjoy immediately!

• • • • • • •

TIP: *You can substitute coconut oil, butter, or olive oil for the ghee in this recipe.*

Toast with Matcha Coconut Butter and Matcha Balsamic Strawberry Compote

MAKES 2 SERVINGS

For the Matcha Coconut Butter:
MAKES ½ CUP

2 cups coconut flakes

1 teaspoon matcha green
tea powder

pinch of sea salt

For the Matcha Balsamic Strawberry Compote:
MAKES 1 CUP

2 cups fresh strawberries,
hulled and chopped

1 tablespoon balsamic
vinegar

2 tablespoons orange juice

1 teaspoon matcha green
tea powder

For the toast:

2 slices sprouted grain
bread

2 tablespoons Matcha
Coconut Butter

2 tablespoons Matcha
Balsamic Strawberry
Compote

To make the Matcha Coconut Butter:

Add the coconut flakes to a large food processor. Process until oils start to release from the coconut flakes and the mixture starts sticking to the bottom and sides of the processor. Stop every minute or two to push the mixture back down toward the blade. Continue for about 6 minutes, or until the mixture is well-combined and watery. Add the matcha powder and salt and pulse to combine. Use immediately or cool to room temperature (it will turn into a solid). The mixture does not have to be refrigerated.

To make the Matcha Balsamic Strawberry Compote:
In a small pot over medium heat, add the strawberries, balsamic vinegar, and orange juice. Stir often, mashing the strawberries as you stir. The liquid will reduce slightly and the strawberries will soften and become more watery. Cook for 8 to 10 minutes. Stir in the matcha powder and remove from the heat.

To make the toast:
Toast the bread to desired crispiness in a toaster or 350°F oven. Spread 1 tablespoon of coconut butter onto each slice of toast and top with 1 tablespoon of the strawberry compote. Enjoy immediately.

Italian Matcha Scramble

• •

MAKES 4 (4-OUNCE) SERVINGS

2 tablespoons extra virgin olive oil

1 small bulb fennel, thinly sliced (about 1½ cups)

¼ cup large red onion, thinly sliced

8 large eggs

½ cup milk

2 tablespoons matcha green tea powder

¼ teaspoon sea salt

cracked black pepper, to taste

½ cup cherry tomatoes, halved

2 large garlic cloves, minced

1 teaspoon chile pepper flakes

¼ cup fresh basil chiffonade, divided

2 tablespoons fresh chopped parsley

2 tablespoons shredded Parmigiano Reggiano cheese or other shredded dry, sharp cheese (optional)

Heat the oil in a large sauté pan over medium heat, then add the fennel and onion. Sauté, stirring every minute or so, until the fennel and onion start to caramelize and take on hint of a brown, about 8 to 10 minutes.

In a separate bowl, combine the eggs, milk, and matcha powder and whisk well. Season with salt and pepper and set aside.

Add the tomatoes, garlic, and chile pepper flakes to the sauté pan. Pour the egg mixture into the sauté pan of veggies, stirring often. Stir in the herbs and cook the mixture until the eggs are no longer runny, about 4 to 5 minutes. Divide among 4 plates and serve immediately, topping each serving with shredded cheese, if using.

• • • • • • •

TIPS: *You can use ghee, butter, or coconut oil instead of olive oil, if you prefer. Additionally, any kind of milk will work, too.*

LUNCH AND SNACKS

One of the challenges with matcha green tea powder is to utilize it in savory dishes where it doesn't overtake the rest of the dish's ingredients. The following section is a mixture of some extremely easy dishes to prepare and some recipes that may take up to two days to complete. Remember to have fun while experimenting with new recipes and include your family as your taste testers so they become more open to trying new things. You never know when you may find your family's next "go-to" meal or snack!

Edamame Matcha Dip

MAKES 4 SERVINGS

2 cups frozen, shelled, unsalted edamame beans

4 cups filtered water

1 tablespoon white miso paste

2 teaspoons sesame oil

1 teaspoon matcha green tea powder

pinch of cracked black pepper

chopped green onion or chopped cilantro, for garnish (optional)

Bring the shelled beans to a boil in the 4 cups water. Reduce heat and simmer for about 5 minutes, or until the edamame is soft and cooked through. Drain the edamame, then add to the bowl of a food processor with all of the ingredients except for the green onion or cilantro. Process until smooth, adding water if a thinner consistency is desired. Garnish with the green onion or cilantro, if using.

TIPS: *Fermented foods such as the miso paste in this recipe are filled with probiotics, which help promote the growth of "good" bacteria in the stomach lining. A strong stomach lining leads to an improved immune system, better absorption of nutrients, and better digestion. Serve with raw vegetables such as carrots, celery, radishes, cauliflower, or whole-grain pita chips. This dip is a great substitute for mayonnaise in wraps and sandwiches.*

Sage Pistachio Matcha Pesto

MAKES 1½ TO 2 CUPS

1 cup raw, shelled pistachios

¼ cup fresh sage leaves

¼ cup fresh parsley

4 large garlic cloves, peeled

⅓ cup extra virgin olive oil

¼ cup filtered water

2 tablespoons lemon juice

1 teaspoon matcha green tea powder

Combine all of the ingredients in a food processor and pulse or process until smooth, adding more water for a thinner consistency.

TIP: *Dollop this pesto atop your favorite soup, use it to dress a grain salad, serve it as a dip with roasted vegetables, or spread it onto your favorite grilled meat.*

Arugula Pesto
• • • • • • • • • • • • • • • • •
MAKES 2 CUPS

4 cups arugula

¾ cup pine nuts

4 large garlic cloves, peeled

¼ cup balsamic vinegar

1 cup extra virgin olive oil

1 teaspoon matcha green tea powder

1 teaspoon sea salt

cracked black pepper, to taste

Combine all of the ingredients in a blender or food processor and blend until a smooth paste forms. Tamp or scrape the sides as needed. Use immediately. Or, store covered in the fridge for a week or in the freezer for up to a month.

• • • • • •
TIP: *Toss your favorite raw or roasted vegetables in this pesto, or spread it on a sandwich, in a wrap, or on grilled meat.*

Green Gazpacho

● ● ● ● ● ● ● ● ● ● ● ● ● ● ● ● ● ● ●

MAKES 4 (8-OUNCE) SERVINGS

½ cup raw almonds

2 small English cucumbers, cut into 1-inch-thick pieces

½ large green bell pepper, cut into large pieces

1 small shallot, cut into thirds

¼ cup fresh parsley

2 tablespoons fresh mint

3 large garlic cloves, smashed

⅔ cup extra virgin olive oil, divided

cracked black pepper, to taste

1 tablespoon matcha green tea powder

½ teaspoon sea salt

To soak the almonds, place them in a small bowl and add water until they are just covered. Allow to soak for at least 4 hours, or overnight. Add the soaked almonds along with the cucumbers, bell pepper, shallot, parsley, mint, garlic, and ⅓ cup of the olive oil to a food processor or blender. Blend on high until the mixture is smooth. Change speed to low and slowly drizzle in the remaining oil to thicken the gazpacho, and season with salt and pepper. Add the matcha powder to the blender right at the end to incorporate. Serve immediately or chill for 30 minutes and serve cold.

● ● ● ● ● ● ●

TIPS: *Substitute the parsley and mint with others of your favorite fresh herbs. Good options include cilantro, basil, chives, and/or dill. You can also add extra-ripe tomatoes, watermelon chunks, or halved grapes to the gazpacho for texture and additional antioxidants.*

Matcha Falafel Pitas with Matcha Tahini Sauce

MAKES ABOUT 24 (1-INCH) FALAFELS

For the falafel pitas:

2 cups dried chickpeas, picked through and rinsed

filtered water

1 tablespoon cumin seeds

1 tablespoon coriander seeds

1 teaspoon baking powder

1 small shallot, coarsely chopped

6 garlic cloves, smashed

¼ teaspoon chile pepper flakes

2 handfuls fresh parsley, coarsely chopped

1 handful fresh cilantro, coarsely chopped

1 handful fresh mint, coarsely chopped

kosher salt and freshly ground black pepper, to taste

coconut oil, for frying, enough to go 1 inch up the sides of the frying pan

8 warm pita breads

Matcha Tahini Sauce

shredded romaine lettuce, sliced tomatoes, chopped cucumbers, and thinly sliced red onion, to top

For the Matcha Tahini Sauce:
MAKES ABOUT 1 CUP

½ cup tahini

½ cup water

juice from 1 lemon

2 garlic cloves, chopped

1 teaspoon matcha green tea powder

pinch of sea salt

pinch of cracked black pepper

To make the falafel pitas:

Split the dried chickpeas between two large glass containers and add filtered, cool water to cover them by at least 2 inches. Soak the beans in the refrigerator for 18 to 24 hours. The chickpeas will swell significantly, so keep an eye on them and add water as necessary. After 18 to 24 hours, drain and rinse them thoroughly.

To toast the cumin and coriander seeds, heat a dry skillet over medium heat. Once hot, add the seeds and toast, shaking the skillet occasionally. Toast until fragrant, then immediately remove from heat. Grind in a spice grinder, or by hand with a mortar and pestle.

Place the rehydrated chickpeas in the bowl of a food processor and pulse to a coarse grind. Don't grind to a smooth paste, but just to the point that there are no whole chickpeas remaining. Add the baking powder, shallot, garlic, cumin, coriander, chile pepper flakes, and herbs; process until the mixture is smooth and well-combined, but not as thick as a paste, scraping down the sides of the bowl as needed. The end result should look fluffy, not pasty and dense. Season with the salt and pepper. Transfer to a bowl and refrigerate for about 15 minutes while completing the next step. (Paste can be made up to a day ahead.)

In a large skillet, add enough coconut oil so that it goes up about 1 inch on the side of the pan. Heat the oil until it reaches about 375°F. To test the oil, put a small amount of the chickpea mixture into the oil and see how quickly it cooks. It should sizzle and brown immediately.

Using a small ice cream scoop or spoon to scoop the falafel mixture, roll the mixture into spheres the size of ping-pong balls. Be careful not to make the balls too tight. Carefully place a few balls at a time into the pan of hot oil, making sure they don't stick to the bottom and they are not overcrowded (adding too many will lower the temperature of your oil and they will not brown). Fry until the chickpea fritters are a crusty dark brown on all sides, turning as needed, about 5 minutes per batch. Remove the falafels with a slotted spoon and drain on a platter lined with paper towels. Season with sea salt as soon as they come out of the oil and onto the platter.

To make the Matcha Tahini Sauce:
Combine all the ingredients in a bowl and whisk until well-combined. Adjust seasoning to taste.

To serve:
Fill warmed pitas with a few falafel balls and a dollop of Matcha Tahini Sauce, then top with lettuce, tomatoes, cucumbers, and red onions.

OPTION: *Serve falafel balls as an appetizer with Matcha Tahini Sauce for dipping, or on top of a salad of mixed greens and fresh veggies, using the Matcha Tahini Sauce as a dressing.*

TIP: *If your food processor is on the small side, split the mixture into smaller batches for best results.*

"Creamed" Spinach and Kale

MAKES 2 (¾-CUP) SERVINGS

2 cups spinach

2½ cups kale, stems removed and chopped

1 teaspoon coconut oil

1 large garlic clove, minced

½ medium yellow onion, chopped

1 teaspoon gluten-free flour

1 cup canned coconut milk

1 teaspoon matcha green tea powder

⅛ teaspoon ground nutmeg

1 teaspoon sea salt

cracked black pepper, to taste

½ teaspoon fresh lemon juice

2 teaspoons nutritional yeast (optional)

⅛ teaspoon chile pepper flakes (optional)

Fill a large pot with 1 inch of water and bring to a boil. Add spinach and kale and simmer until withered. Quickly remove from the heat, pour into a colander, and rinse under cold water to stop cooking. Grab the greens by the handful and squeeze out the excess water from the leaves, then place on a cutting board and chop the mixture well.

In a small saucepan on medium heat, melt the coconut oil. Add the garlic and onion, and cook just until soft. Add the gluten-free flour, stirring to form a paste. Slowly whisk in the coconut milk and cook until slightly thickened. Whisk in the matcha powder, nutmeg, salt, pepper, and lemon juice, along with the nutritional yeast and chile pepper flakes, if using. Add in the spinach and kale mixture and mix well. Serve immediately.

Beet, Watercress, and Matcha Goat Cheese Salad

● ● ● ● ● ● ● ● ● ● ● ● ● ● ● ● ● ● ● ●
MAKES 4 (6-OUNCE) SALADS

2½ ounces goat cheese, softened

6 medium (3-inch diameter) beets, tops removed and scrubbed

1½ teaspoons matcha green tea powder

1 teaspoon chopped fresh chives

2 loosely packed cups watercress

juice of ½ lemon

2 tablespoons extra virgin olive oil

½ teaspoon sea salt

cracked black pepper, to taste

Take the goat cheese out of the refrigerator so that it can warm to room temperature. Place the scrubbed beets in a small pot, cover with water, and bring to a boil, covered with a lid. Boil for 30 to 40 minutes or until easily pierced with a fork.

While the beets are boiling, combine the goat cheese, matcha powder, and chives in a small bowl and whip with a fork until the matcha is evenly incorporated. Set aside.

Drain the cooked beets in a colander to cool a bit. When cool enough to work with but still warm, slide the skins off the beets under running water. Once peeled, cube the beets. Lightly wash and spin-dry the watercress. Place the beets onto a serving dish, sprinkle with watercress, and use a teaspoon to drop small spoonfuls of the goat cheese mixture on top. Drizzle with lemon juice and olive oil, and sprinkle with salt and cracked black pepper. Serve chilled or at room temperature.

● ● ● ● ● ●
TIP: *If you don't have a salad spinner, rinse the watercress, then lightly press it into a clean kitchen towel to remove as much water as possible.*

Avocado Seaweed Dip

MAKES 1 CUP

2 large avocados, pitted

2 tablespoons extra virgin olive oil

juice from 1 large lime

1 teaspoon sesame oil

1 large garlic clove, peeled

1 teaspoon matcha green tea powder

¼ teaspoon sea salt

2 teaspoons kelp flakes, plus ¼ teaspoon for garnish

1 to 2 teaspoons Sriracha hot sauce, for garnish (optional)

fresh vegetables, chips, or pita bread, to serve

Combine all ingredients except ¼ teaspoon kelp flakes and the Sriracha in a large food processor or blender. Process or blend until smooth. Chill for at least 30 minutes before serving, then sprinkle the kelp flakes and drizzle the Sriracha hot sauce on top, if using. Serve with fresh vegetables, chips, or pita bread.

Heirloom Tomato Salad with Matcha Sesame Dressing

MAKES 2 SERVINGS

For the salad:

1 large heirloom tomato, chopped, or several mini heirloom tomatoes

pinch of sea salt

1 teaspoon finely chopped chives

For the Matcha Sesame Dressing:
MAKES 1 CUP

¼ cup orange juice

2 tablespoons rice wine vinegar

1 large garlic clove, peeled

2 tablespoons fresh ginger, peeled and chopped

¾ teaspoon matcha green tea powder

¼ teaspoon ground mustard

4 tablespoons sesame oil

6 tablespoons extra virgin olive oil

½ teaspoon sea salt, or to taste

2 tablespoons black sesame seeds

To make the salad:

Wash the tomato(es) well and cut into thin wedges.

To make the Matcha Sesame Dressing:

Add the orange juice, vinegar, garlic, and ginger to a small bowl. Using an immersion blender or a handheld whisk, blend or whisk until incorporated. Add the matcha powder and mustard, then slowly start adding the oils in a thin, steady stream until the mixture emulsifies and thickens. If it is too thick, add a sprinkle of water or orange juice. Season with salt and transfer to a bowl, then stir in the sesame seeds so they remain whole.

To serve:

Divide the tomatoes between 2 plates, then drizzle each with 1 to 2 tablespoons of dressing and a pinch of sea salt and chopped chives. Serve immediately.

• • • • • •

TIP: *Use this dressing to accompany your favorite Asian-inspired salad or veggies, or as a marinade for grilled meats.*

Grilled Portobellos with Matcha Chimichurri

· ·

MAKES 4 SERVINGS

For the grilled portobellos:

4 tablespoons extra virgin olive oil

3 tablespoons balsamic vinegar

½ teaspoon matcha green tea powder

½ teaspoon sea salt

⅛ teaspoon cracked black pepper

4 large portobello mushrooms, stems and gills removed

½ cup Matcha Chimichurri

For the Matcha Chimichurri:

MAKES ABOUT 8 OUNCES

¼ cup fresh chopped parsley

¼ cup fresh chopped cilantro

1 tablespoon fresh chopped mint

2 tablespoons chopped oregano

4 large garlic cloves, minced

1 teaspoon capers in brine, drained

¼ teaspoon sea salt

¼ teaspoon cracked black pepper

½ teaspoon chile pepper flakes (optional)

3 tablespoons red wine vinegar

½ cup extra virgin olive oil

Prepare the mushrooms. In a small bowl, combine the olive oil, balsamic vinegar, matcha powder, salt, and pepper. Pour over the portobellos and allow to marinate for at least 30 minutes, flipping at least once.

While they marinate, make the Matcha Chimichurri. Combine the parsley, cilantro, mint, oregano, garlic, and capers in a bowl, then add the salt, black pepper, and chile pepper flakes, if using. Stir in the red wine vinegar and olive oil and allow to sit at least 30 minutes before serving. Chimichurri can be made the day before and refrigerated overnight.

Heat a grill pan over high heat. Place the marinated portobellos on the hot grill pan and grill for 3 minutes per side, or until grill marks show. Remove from the pan after cooking both sides and slice into ¼-inch-thick slices. Place sliced mushrooms on a plate and drizzle each mushroom with 2 tablespoons of the chimichurri. Serve warm or chilled.

Indian Spiced Lentils with Matcha Yogurt

MAKES 4 TO 6 (12-OUNCE) SERVINGS

For the spiced lentils:

2 cups green lentils

1 teaspoon coriander seeds

1 teaspoon cumin seeds

1 to 2 tablespoons ghee

1 teaspoon ground cinnamon

1½ teaspoons ground turmeric

1 small onion, chopped

3 garlic cloves, minced

1-inch piece ginger, peeled and minced (about 2 tablespoons)

1 (15-ounce) can diced tomatoes, no salt added

6 cups vegetable broth

1 to 2 tablespoons sea salt, or to taste

1 tablespoon matcha green tea powder

cilantro leaves, for garnish (optional)

For the Matcha Yogurt:

1½ teaspoons matcha green tea powder

½ cup full-fat yogurt

Do ahead:

Place the 2 cups lentils into a medium bowl. Cover with filtered water and soak for 1 to 2 hours. Drain lentils in a small colander and rinse well. Set aside.

To make the Matcha Yogurt:

Whisk the matcha green tea powder into the yogurt. Place in the refrigerator until you're ready to serve the lentils.

To make the spiced lentils:

Heat a small pan on high heat without oil. Add the coriander and cumin seeds to the hot pan, shaking often until the spices are fragrant, 2 to 3 minutes. Remove the seeds from the pan immediately and use a spice grinder to grind until smooth. Set aside.

Heat a large pot over medium heat. Add the ghee, freshly ground spices, cinnamon, turmeric, and onion. Cook for 2 minutes, then add the garlic and ginger and cook an additional 3 to 4 minutes, stirring often, until the onion is translucent. Add the tomatoes, then the lentils and broth. Cover and simmer over low heat for 40 to 50 minutes. Add salt to taste. Stir the matcha powder in right before serving. Serve hot with a dollop of the Matcha Yogurt and a cilantro leaf for garnish.

• • • • • •

TIPS. *While this recipe calls for green lentils, you can using any color! Lentils should be rinsed and soaked for up to an hour before cooking, depending on the type of lentil. Soaking cuts down the cooking time and also makes them easier to digest. Also, you can swap coconut oil for the ghee in this recipe, if you prefer.*

Candied Matcha Carrots

● ●

MAKES 2 (8-OUNCE) SERVINGS

3 large carrots, peeled and cut diagonally into ½-inch-thick pieces, about 3 cups

½ teaspoon ground cinnamon

1½ teaspoons matcha green tea powder

2 teaspoons coconut palm sugar

½ teaspoon sea salt

1 tablespoon avocado oil

Preheat the oven to 375°F. In a medium bowl, combine all of the ingredients and toss until the carrots are coated evenly. Spread carrots in a thin layer on a parchment-lined cookie sheet. Place the cookie sheet in the center rack of the oven and roast for about 15 minutes or until carrots are tender and the sugar has caramelized. Serve immediately, or chill to add to a salad of grains or greens.

● ● ● ● ● ● ●

TIP: *Don't have avocado oil on hand? You can use extra virgin olive oil or melted coconut oil, too.*

Cauliflower and Snap Pea Stir-Fry

· · · · · · · · · · · · · · ·

MAKES 4 (¾-CUP) SERVINGS

½ teaspoon sesame oil

1 teaspoon coconut oil

⅛ teaspoon chile pepper flakes

2 teaspoons fresh ginger, peeled and minced

4 cups small cauliflower florets (1 small cauliflower head)

½ cup onion, cut in half and thinly sliced

1½ cups snap peas, cut diagonally into ½-inch wide pieces

2 large garlic cloves, minced

1 tablespoon tamari or soy sauce

1½ teaspoon matcha green tea powder

black sesame seeds, for garnish (optional)

Heat a large sauté pan on medium heat and add the sesame oil and the coconut oil to melt. Once the oil is hot, add the chile pepper flakes, ginger, and cauliflower in a thin, even layer. Cook the cauliflower for 4 to 5 minutes, stirring occasionally. Add the onion and snap peas and cook an additional 3 to 4 minutes, or until the onion is translucent and the snap peas have browned a bit. Finish by adding the garlic and sautéing an additional 1 to 2 minutes. Add the tamari and matcha green tea and toss well. Serve hot and garnish with black sesame seeds.

· · · · · ·

TIP: *Tamari is a wheat-free alternative to soy sauce.*

Honey, Sriracha, and Matcha-Glazed Salmon

MAKES 2 (3-OUNCE) SERVINGS

2 (3-ounce) salmon filets

2 tablespoons raw honey

1 teaspoon Sriracha hot sauce

1 teaspoon matcha green tea powder

½ teaspoon sea salt

Preheat the oven to 400°F. Remove the filets from refrigerator and let the fish come to room temperature.

Meanwhile, in a small bowl, combine the honey, Sriracha, matcha powder, and salt and whisk well until there are no lumps. Spread the mixture over the salmon filets and rub the mixture into both sides of each filet. Place the filets onto a baking sheet lined with parchment paper at least 3 inches apart from each other, then place in the middle rack of your preheated oven. Roast for 12 to 14 minutes or until the edges are flaky and the center is still slightly underdone. Remove from the baking sheet and let them rest about 2 minutes to allow them to continue to cook through. Enjoy hot or cool and shred to add to your favorite salad or sandwich.

Matcha Green Goddess Dip

• •

MAKES 2 CUPS

2 tablespoons fresh chopped parsley

2 tablespoons fresh chopped chives

2 tablespoons fresh chopped tarragon

2 tablespoons fresh chopped basil

2 tablespoons chopped, peeled shallot

¾ cup whole Greek yogurt

3 to 4 anchovy filets (about 3 ounces)

1 tablespoon matcha green tea powder

¼ cup lemon juice

½ cup filtered water (more or less depending on desired consistency)

1 teaspoon sea salt, or to taste

cracked black pepper, to taste

Prior to chopping the fresh herbs, remove the thick stems and then rough chop the tops of the stems with the leaves. Combine all of the ingredients, except the salt and pepper, in a blender or food processor and blend until smooth. Season the dressing with salt and pepper. Cover and chill at least 30 minutes before serving. Can be made a day ahead. Serve drizzled over mixed greens, as a mayonnaise substitute, or as a dip.

• • • • • •

TIPS: *For a more rustic look to this dressing, the herbs and anchovies can be chopped by hand and combined in a mixing bowl instead of the blender. Watch the salt if you love anchovies! Anchovies are packed with salt so if you go heavy on them, watch how much additional salt, you add in this recipe. Also, the longer the mixture sits, the more the flavors develop. Taste the mix right before serving to see if it does really need more salt.*

Matcha and Kelp Popcorn

MAKES 10 TO 12 CUPS

For the popcorn:

4 tablespoons coconut oil

⅓ cup popcorn kernels

For the seasoning:

6 tablespoons unsalted butter

3 tablespoons kelp flakes

1½ tablespoons matcha green tea powder

1 tablespoon sesame seeds

2 teaspoons salt

To make the popcorn:

In a large, heavy-bottomed pot, melt the coconut oil over medium-high heat so that it coats the bottom of the pan. Add the popcorn, coat with oil, cover, and cook over medium-high heat. When the kernels start to pop, carefully shake the pot with the lid on until the popping slows to a few seconds between each pop. Shaking the pot often will help to prevent the popcorn from burning. Popping all the corn should take about 4 to 5 minutes, depending on how hot your stove and pot get.

Pour the popped popcorn into an extra-large mixing bowl, or multiple bowls.

To make the seasoning:

In a small saucepan, melt the butter on low heat and add the kelp flakes, matcha powder, sesame seeds, and salt, stirring to combine. Drizzle this over the popcorn and toss well. Serve warm or at room temperature.

• • • • • •

TIP: *The kelp flakes in this recipe can be replaced with furikake, togarashi, or any other Asian spice blend that contains seaweed. Seaweed is a potent superfood that adds extra minerals and vitamins to many foods.*

DESSERT

· · · · · · · · · · ·

For the following recipes matcha has been incorporated into an array of desserts and baked goods for its vibrant color and bold but yet subtle flavor! From the basic muffins and cookies to the more complicated puddings and ice creams, matcha is a very easy ingredient to add to most recipes. The biggest tips to making great matcha desserts is to not add too much and knowing how to add the matcha powder.

Because of its unique flavor in sweets, matcha should be used in moderation. Too much can create an off-putting grassy flavor. While it packs a punch of flavor on its own, matcha pairs very well with other popular flavors such as chocolate (white, milk, and dark), oranges, raspberries, and coconut, to name a few.

When adding matcha to any recipe, especially desserts, it is very important to add the matcha powder to the dry ingredients or to the liquid ingredients. This is an essential step because it will eliminate any potential lumps and to ensure that the matcha powder has been fully incorporated with the other ingredients. When adding the matcha powder to the dry ingredients, use a whisk to combine, whisking until it's well blended. When adding the matcha powder to the liquid ingredients, avoid mixing it with eggs, but milks (whole, soy, almond, etc.) and creams are ideal. If the recipes require you to heat the liquid or bring to a boil, then whisk in the matcha powder after, not before. Heating can intensify the flavor of the green tea, which can result in a bitter and grassy taste.

The following dessert recipes were created by Chef Lasheeda Perry, a contributing author to this collection of recipes!

Matcha Panna Cotta

MAKES 11 (½-CUP) SERVINGS

1 cup whole milk, divided

3 cups heavy cream

2 envelopes (2½ teaspoons) gelatin

2 teaspoons vanilla extract

1 cup grade A maple syrup

2 tablespoons, plus 1 teaspoon matcha green tea powder

seasonal fruit, to garnish (optional)

Pour ½ cup of the milk into a small pot and sprinkle the gelatin over it. Allow the mixture to sit for 10 minutes.

Meanwhile, combine the remainder of the milk with the heavy cream, vanilla extract, and maple syrup in a medium saucepan and cook over medium-low heat. Whisk in the matcha powder and bring the mixture to a simmer.

Place the gelatin-milk mixture on low heat until the gelatin dissolves. Using a whisk, gradually add the gelatin-milk mixture to the simmering heavy cream mixture. Once fully incorporated, strain the mixture through a fine-mesh strainer into a bowl. Immediately pour the strained mixture into 11 (4-ounce) ramekins or dishes. Refrigerate the panna cotta for a minimum of 2 hours before serving, or overnight. Serve chilled as is, or topped with sliced seasonal fruit.

Gluten-Free Matcha Muffin

MAKES 10 TO 12 MUFFINS

1½ cups gluten-free flour

½ teaspoon ground cinnamon

1½ teaspoons plus ⅛ teaspoon baking powder

¾ cup plus 2 tablespoons light brown sugar

1 teaspoon vanilla extract

¼ cup heavy cream

¾ cup plus 2 tablespoons soy milk

1 tablespoon matcha green tea powder

2 eggs

7 tablespoons unsalted butter, melted

Preheat the oven to 350°F. In a large bowl, mix the gluten-free flour, cinnamon, baking powder, and brown sugar. In a medium pot, combine the vanilla extract, heavy cream, and soy milk. Heat to 98°F, as measured by a thermometer. Remove the pot from the heat and whisk in the matcha powder. Using a stand mixer with the paddle attachment, combine the dry and wet ingredients, including the eggs and melted butter. Mix on speed 2 for 1 minute. Scrape the sides and bottom of the bowl. Mix batter again on speed 2 for an additional 30 seconds.

Line a muffin tin with paper liners and fill each three-quarters full with batter. Bake in a preheated oven for 15 to 20 minutes. The muffins are done once an inserted toothpick comes out clean.

Cool muffins completely before serving. Store in an airtight container at room temperature for up to a week.

TIP: *Chef Lasheeda's favorite gluten-free flour is Cup4Cup.*

Brown Sugar Matcha Marshmallows

• • • • • • • • • • • • • • • •

MAKES 8 TO 10 (2 TO 3 PIECE) SERVINGS

3 envelopes (7½ teaspoons) gelatin

1 cup cold water, divided

1½ cups light brown sugar

1 cup organic non-GMO corn syrup

¼ teaspoon salt

½ teaspoon vanilla extract

4 teaspoons matcha green tea powder

Place the gelatin and half of the cold water in the bowl of a stand mixer fitted with a whisk attachment. Meanwhile, combine the remainder of the water, brown sugar, corn syrup, and salt in a medium saucepan. Place the saucepan over medium heat and cook to 240°F, as measured by a candy thermometer. Once that temperature is reached, immediately remove it from the heat.

Return to the gelatin-water mixture. Turn the mixer on to speed 1. While actively mixing, gradually pour the sugar syrup into the gelatin mixture. Avoid touching the whisk if possible. Increase the speed to 4. Whip until the bowl feels lukewarm, 10 to 12 minutes. During the last 2 minutes, reduce the speed to 1, then gradually add the vanilla extract and matcha powder.

Lightly coat a 9 x 13-inch baking pan with baking spray. Pour the marshmallow mixture into the prepared pan. Using an oiled rubber spatula, evenly spread the marshmallow throughout the pan.

Allow the marshmallows to set, uncovered, overnight.

Flip the marshmallows onto a cutting board. Lightly oil a pizza cutter and cut the marshmallows into evenly sized pieces, such as 1-inch cubes or 2-inch bars. Keep the marshmallows stored in an airtight container for up to 3 days.

Matcha Rice Pudding

· ·

MAKES 15 (½-CUP) SERVINGS

2 cups water

3½ cups whole milk

2½ tablespoons matcha green tea powder

2 cinnamon sticks

¼ teaspoon salt

1 vanilla bean

2 teaspoons grated orange zest

1¼ cups grade A maple syrup

1 cup medium-grain white rice

½ cup golden raisins

In a medium saucepan, combine the water and milk. Whisk in the matcha powder. Add the cinnamon sticks, salt, vanilla bean, orange zest, and maple syrup. Bring to a boil over medium-low heat. Stir in the rice and cook, uncovered, for approximately 30 minutes. Stir occasionally. Add the golden raisins and simmer for an additional 10 to 15 minutes. Stir regularly. Remove from heat and pour into a ceramic dish. Cool rice pudding for 2 hours to room temperature. Keep covered and stir occasionally while cooling. The rice pudding will thicken as it cools. Once cooled, serve immediately.

· · · · · · ·

TIPS: *Leftover pudding can be refrigerated for up to 1 week. It will continue to thicken when chilled, so just add a little maple syrup and milk until desired consistency is achieved. Also, golden raisins can be replaced with other dried fruit such as cranberries, currants, or cherries.*

Warm Coconut Green Tea Tapioca Pudding

MAKES 4 (½-CUP) SERVINGS

½ cup shredded unsweetened coconut

1 cup whole milk

1 cup canned coconut milk

¼ cup small tapioca pearls

¼ cup light brown sugar, divided

½ teaspoon vanilla extract

pinch of salt

½ teaspoon grated orange zest

2¼ teaspoons matcha green tea powder

1 egg yolk

toasted coconut, for garnish

Preheat the oven to 325°F. Place the shredded coconut onto a baking sheet and bake, shaking the pan occasionally, until the coconut is light golden brown.

In a medium saucepan, combine the whole milk, coconut milk, tapioca pearls, half of the brown sugar, vanilla extract, salt, and orange zest. Over medium-low heat, bring the mixture to a boil, stirring constantly. Reduce the heat to low and gradually stir in the matcha powder. Cook for an additional 5 minutes, stirring constantly.

Meanwhile, in a small bowl, combine the remaining brown sugar with the egg yolk and whisk well. Whisk 1 cup of the hot milk mixture into the yolk mixture, then add it back to the tapioca until well combined.

Bring the tapioca to a gentle simmer over low heat. Cook and stir for 2 more minutes or until the pudding becomes thick enough to coat the back of a spoon. Remove from the heat and pour into serving dishes. Garnish with toasted coconut.

Gluten-Free Chocolate Chip Matcha Pancakes

MAKES 6 PANCAKES

1 cup gluten-free flour

2 tablespoons light brown sugar

2 teaspoons baking powder

½ teaspoon salt

pinch of ground nutmeg

1 tablespoon matcha green tea powder

½ teaspoon vanilla extract

1 cup whole milk

1 egg

2 tablespoons unsalted butter, melted

1½ tablespoons unsalted butter

1½ tablespoons coconut oil

½ cup bittersweet chocolate chips

maple syrup, for serving

In a medium bowl, combine the gluten-free flour, brown sugar, baking powder, salt, nutmeg, and matcha powder and mix well.

In a separate medium bowl, whisk together the vanilla extract, milk, egg, and melted butter and mix well.

Add the dry ingredients to the milk mixture and whisk until it just begins to incorporate. Do not overmix it; the batter should have some small lumps.

Heat a large, nonstick pan with ½ tablespoon of butter and oil each. For each pancake, spoon 4 tablespoons of batter onto the pan. Cook 2 pancakes at a time.

Sprinkle approximately 1 tablespoon of chocolate chips per pancake. Cook until the surface of the pancake begins to bubble and burst. Flip the pancakes over and cook for an additional 2 minutes. Transfer the pancakes to a platter.

Add another ½ tablespoon of oil and butter and continue cooking pancakes with the remaining batter. Serve immediately with maple syrup.

Gluten-Free Matcha Cranberry White Chocolate Chip Scones

MAKES 12 SCONES

2 teaspoons matcha green tea powder

1¼ cup heavy cream, divided

2 cups gluten-free flour, plus ½ cup for dusting

⅓ cup brown sugar

2 teaspoons baking powder

1 teaspoon grated orange zest

½ teaspoon salt

½ cup (1 stick) cold unsalted butter

1 cup dried cranberries

1 cup mini white chocolate chips

pinch of salt

Preheat the oven to 350°F. In a small bowl, whisk the matcha powder into ¾ cup of the heavy cream.

In a medium bowl, combine the gluten-free flour, brown sugar, baking powder, orange zest, and salt.

Chop the butter into 1-inch cubes. Add the butter to the dry ingredients. Using a pastry cutter or your hands, cut the butter into the dry ingredients until coarse crumbs are achieved. Add the matcha mixture, but do not fully incorporate. Add the dried cranberries and white chocolate chips. Mix until all of the ingredients have been fully incorporated.

Place the dough on a lightly floured surface (use gluten-free flour for dusting). Using a rolling pin, roll the dough to 1-inch thickness. With a square cookie cutter, cut out the scones close together to avoid excess scraps. The scraps can be re-rolled.

Place the scones 1 inch apart on a parchment-lined baking sheet pan. Combine the remaining ½ cup heavy cream with the salt and brush the tops of the scones with the heavy cream and salt mixture. Bake for 10 to 12 minutes, or until the bottoms of the scones are golden brown. Allow to cool and serve immediately. Store at room temperature in an airtight container for up to 1 week.

Brown Butter Matcha Rice Crispy Treats

MAKES 12 TO 18 SERVINGS

½ cup (1 stick) unsalted butter

9 cups Brown Sugar Matcha Marshmallows (page 73), divided

1 teaspoon vanilla extract

3 teaspoons matcha green tea powder

10 cups crispy rice cereal

Coat a 9 x 13-inch baking pan with cooking spray. Melt the butter in a large pot over medium heat. As the butter melts, stir occasionally. The butter will start to bubble and foam, which is normal. As the foam begins to subside and the butter begins to brown, keep stirring and keep a close eye on it. Once it's deep brown in color immediately turn off the heat. The residual heat will be used for the remainder of this recipe.

Stir in 8 cups of the marshmallows and mix until about 75 percent of the marshmallows have melted. Add the vanilla extract and matcha powder. Pour in the cereal and quickly stir until the crispy rice is fully covered with the marshmallow mixture. Quickly stir in the last cup of marshmallows. Do not allow them to melt completely but to be marbled throughout the crispy rice. Immediately pour the mixture into the prepared pan. Evenly spread the mixture throughout the pan. Allow treats to cool for 4 hours, then remove from pan and cut into desired size.

Matcha Chia Seed Pudding

MAKES 4 (½-CUP) SERVINGS

2½ cups almond milk

2 teaspoons matcha green tea powder

½ teaspoon vanilla extract

4 tablespoons agave nectar

pinch of ground nutmeg

½ teaspoon grated orange zest

½ cup chia seeds

¼ cup sliced almonds, toasted, for garnish

½ cup orange segments, for garnish

In a large mason jar, combine the almond milk, matcha powder, vanilla extract, agave nectar, nutmeg, and orange zest. Lid the jar and shake very well to combine the ingredients. Add the chia seeds and shake very well again. Refrigerate the jar overnight, shaking 3 to 4 times. The mixture should thicken like a pudding.

The next day, distribute the pudding among four dishes. Garnish the puddings with the toasted almonds and orange segments and serve.

Matcha Pavlova

· ·

MAKES 8 (1-SLICE) SERVINGS

4 egg whites

1¼ cups light brown sugar

1 teaspoon vanilla extract

2 tablespoons matcha
green tea powder

Matcha Whipped Cream
(page 88), for garnish

3 cups seasonal berries,
for garnish

Preheat the oven to 275°F. Using a 9-inch round cake pan as a guide, trace the perimeter of the pan onto parchment paper. Place the parchment paper onto a baking sheet pan.

Fill a medium saucepan three-quarters full with water and bring to a boil. Turn off the heat. Set up a double boiler by resting a bowl comfortably on top of the pot. Place the egg whites and brown sugar in the bowl. Whisk constantly until the mixture is warm to the touch and the sugar has dissolved. Using a hand mixer, whip on high speed until the mixture is fluffy and glossy. Reduce the speed to low and add the vanilla extract, then the matcha powder. Mix for 1 additional minute, or until the matcha powder has been fully incorporated.

Use a spatula to pour the meringue in the center of the 9-inch circle you drew on the parchment paper. Use the spatula to evenly spread the meringue out toward the edges. Bake for 1 hour and 20 minutes, then turn off the oven but keep the meringue in the oven. Once the meringue is completely dry, it can be removed from the oven. Allow the meringue to cool. Once cool, topped with matcha whipped cream and seasonal berries and serve.

Toasted Coconut and Matcha Ice Cream

• • • • • • • • • • • • • • • • • • • •

MAKES 4 (½-CUP) SERVINGS

½ cup shredded coconut

1 cup coconut milk

1 cup skim milk

½ cup evaporated milk

½ cup, plus 2 tablespoons brown sugar

½ vanilla bean and seeds

pinch of salt

2 tablespoons matcha green tea powder

Preheat oven to 325°F. Spread the shredded coconut onto a baking sheet and bake for approximately 4 minutes, or until it's golden brown, occasionally stirring to ensure that it bakes evenly. Meanwhile, in a medium saucepan, combine the milks, brown sugar, vanilla bean and seeds, and salt, then stir in the toasted coconut. Bring the mixture to a boil and remove from heat. Cover the top of the pot with plastic wrap and allow the mixture to steep at room temperature for 30 minutes.

After 30 minutes, bring the mixture to a second boil, then reduce the heat to low. Whisk in the matcha powder until it's completely dissolved. Strain the mixture through a fine-mesh strainer into a separate bowl. Cool the mixture by placing the bowl into a larger bowl that's filled with ice and water (an ice bath). Occasionally stir the ice cream base so that a skin doesn't form. Once the ice cream base is cool, follow the directions of your ice cream maker and mix. Allow the ice cream to solidify in the freezer for at least 3 hours before serving.

Dark Chocolate Matcha Truffles

MAKES 24 TRUFFLES

¼ cup heavy cream

1 tablespoon unsalted butter

⅔ cup chopped semisweet chocolate

¼ cup matcha green tea powder

In a small saucepan, combine the heavy cream and butter over medium heat and bring to a simmer. Add the chopped chocolate to the scalded cream and whisk until smooth. Pour the mixture into a bowl. Cover the bowl very well with plastic wrap and allow to cool to room temperature.

Once the ganache is cooled and set, using a small scoop, scoop balls of the ganache onto a parchment-lined baking sheet. Chill in the refrigerator for 5 minutes.

Roll the balls with your hands into smooth, uniform balls. Dip each ganache ball into the matcha and shake off the excess. Serve at room temperature.

Matcha-Flavored Milk

MAKES 4 (½-CUP) SERVINGS

3 tablespoons matcha green tea powder

¼ vanilla bean

¼ cup light brown sugar

4 cups whole milk

½ teaspoon grated orange zest

Sift the matcha powder into a small bowl. Slice the vanilla bean and scrape the seeds into the brown sugar in a separate bowl. In a saucepan, combine the whole milk, vanilla bean–brown sugar mixture, orange zest, and sifted matcha powder. Bring to a simmer then strain. Refrigerate overnight and serve chilled.

Maple and Matcha Cream Pie

MAKES 10 (1-SLICE) SERVINGS

For the crust:

2½ cups quinoa flakes

⅔ cup almond flour

⅔ cup blanched almonds

¼ cup maple syrup

⅔ cup coconut oil, melted

2 tablespoons water

For the maple and matcha custard:

1½ cups heavy cream

¼ cup maple sugar

1 tablespoon grade A
maple syrup

½ teaspoon vanilla extract

1 tablespoon matcha
green tea powder

2 egg yolks

2 teaspoons powdered
gelatin

¼ cup water

To make the crust:

Preheat the oven to 350°F. Spray a 9-inch pie pan with baking spray. Combine the quinoa flakes, almond flour, and almonds in a food processor for 2 to 3 minutes. Add the maple syrup, then the oil, and mix until it comes together. Add the water and pulse again.

Place the dough into the prepared pie pan, making sure the dough covers the inside of the entire pie pan. Firmly press the dough into the pan. Bake for approximately 15 minutes or until fully baked. Allow the crust to cool completely.

To make the maple and matcha custard:

In a medium saucepan, combine the heavy cream, maple sugar, maple syrup, vanilla extract, and matcha powder and bring to a simmer. Meanwhile, bloom the gelatin by mixing the powdered gelatin with the water. Make sure to mix it very well so that all of the gelatin dissolves. This step will create a smooth and set custard. Allow the gelatin-water mixture to sit for 5 minutes.

Place your egg yolks into a small bowl. Once the cream mixture has come to a simmer, pour ½ cup of the hot liquid into the egg yolks and mix well. Then pour the yolk mixture into the pot of simmering cream. Stir constantly with a rubber spatula or wooden spoon and cook until the mixture coats the back of the spoon.

Remove from the heat and add the bloomed gelatin. Stir until the gelatin has melted completely. Strain the mixture through a fine-mesh strainer, then pour the custard into the baked pie shell, filling it to the top. Refrigerate the entire pie for at least 3 hours, but preferably overnight, and serve chilled.

• • • • • •

TIP: *This pie can be garnished with toasted almonds, Matcha Whipped Cream (page 88), or seasonal berries.*

Grand Marnier Macerated Raspberries with Matcha Whipped Cream

MAKES 4 (½ CUP RASPBERRIES AND 2 TABLESPOONS
OF WHIPPED CREAM) SERVINGS

For the macerated raspberries:

2 cups fresh raspberries

1 tablespoon agave nectar

1 tablespoon Grand Marnier

½ teaspoon grated orange zest

For the Matcha Whipped Cream:

1 cup heavy cream

1 teaspoon matcha green tea powder

3 tablespoons light brown sugar

1 teaspoon vanilla extract

To make the macerated raspberries:

In a medium bowl, toss the fresh raspberries with the agave nectar, Grand Marnier, and orange zest. Place mixture into desired serving dish.

To make the Matcha Whipped Cream:

In a separate bowl, combine the heavy cream and matcha powder. With a hand mixer, whip the mixture until bubbles form. At this point, gradually add the brown sugar and then the vanilla extract. Continue whipping until medium stiff peaks form.

Top the macerated raspberries with the matcha whipped cream. Serve immediately.

• • • • • •
CHEF'S NOTE: *The amount of agave nectar will vary depending on the natural sweetness of the raspberries.*

• • • • • •
TIP: *Matcha whipped cream can be made 1 hour in advance.*

Matcha Almond Chocolate Chip Sable

MAKES 12 SABLES

2 cups almond flour

½ cup light brown sugar

1 teaspoon baking powder

¼ teaspoon salt

1 teaspoon grated orange zest

3 tablespoons coconut oil

2½ teaspoons vanilla extract

½ teaspoon almond extract

2 tablespoons almond milk

4 teaspoons matcha green tea powder

½ cup semisweet chocolate chips

Preheat the oven to 325°F. In a large bowl, combine the almond flour, brown sugar, baking powder, salt, and orange zest. In another bowl, combine the coconut oil, vanilla extract, almond extract, almond milk, and matcha powder, then add this mixture to the almond flour mixture. Mix briefly, then fold in the chocolate chips.

On a parchment-lined baking sheet, portion the dough into small scoops. Make sure to set scoops evenly apart. Bake for 11 to 13 minutes, rotating the baking sheet halfway through the baking process. Allow cookies to cool completely before serving.

Conversion Charts

Volume Conversions

U.S.	U.S. equivalent	Metric
1 tablespoon (3 teaspoons)	½ fluid ounce	15 milliliters
¼ cup	2 fluid ounces	60 milliliters
⅓ cup	3 fluid ounces	90 milliliters
½ cup	4 fluid ounces	120 milliliters
⅔ cup	5 fluid ounces	150 milliliters
¾ cup	6 fluid ounces	180 milliliters
1 cup	8 fluid ounces	240 milliliters
2 cups	16 fluid ounces	480 milliliters

Weight Conversions

U.S.	Metric
½ ounce	15 grams
1 ounce	30 grams
2 ounces	60 grams
¼ pound	115 grams
⅓ pound	150 grams
½ pound	225 grams
¾ pound	350 grams
1 pound	450 grams

Temperature Conversions

Fahrenheit (°F)	Celsius (°C)
200°F	95°C
225°F	110°C
250°F	120°C
275°F	135°C
300°F	150°C
325°F	165°C
350°F	175°C
375°F	190°C
400°F	200°C
425°F	220°C
450°F	230°C

Recipe Index

Acknowledgments

Mariza Snyder: I would love to acknowledge my husband, Alex, for his amazing support and recipe-testing skills. He's my partner in crime. I would also love to thank my coauthors for their incredible teamwork!

Lauren Clum: I'd like to dedicate this book to the newest addition to our family, my baby girl. Additionally, a huge thanks is owed to my amazingly supportive husband, and my brilliant and talented coauthors.

Anna V. Zulaica: I would like to thank my coauthors for being such wonderful and inspiring women. I would also like to thank my family and friends for being supportive and for being the best recipe tasters.

Lasheeda Perry: Of course, I want to thank my family, friends, chef instructors, and anyone else who plays a pivotal role in my career. But, in all honesty, my recipes would not be featured in this book if it weren't for FoodGal. There's amazing hidden potential in all of us, so I truly thank you, FoodGal, for helping me uncover my full potential.

About the Authors

Dr. Mariza Snyder is a passionate and dedicated wellness practitioner and speaker committed to inspiring people to live a healthy and abundant life through plant-based nutrition and simple lifestyle changes. She is the coauthor of *The Low GI Slow Cooker: Delicious and Easy Dishes Made Healthy with the Glycemic Index.* She lives with her husband in Oakland, CA.

Dr. Lauren Clum is a chiropractor committed to helping people recognize their own healing capacities. She is the founder and director of The Specific Chiropractic Center in Oakland, California, and has coauthored several books on health and wellness: *The Antioxidant Counter: A Pocket Guide to the Revolutionary ORAC Scale for Choosing Healthy Foods, The DASH Diet Cookbook: Quick and Delicious Recipes for Losing Weight, Preventing Diabetes, and Lowering Blood Pressure, The Low GI Slow Cooker: Delicious and Easy Dishes Made Healthy with the Glycemic Index,* and *Water Infusions: Refreshing, Detoxifying and Healthy Recipes for Your Home Infuser.* Dr. Clum completed her undergraduate degree in business administration, with an emphasis in management, at Sonoma State University in Rohnert Park, California. After graduating with honors from Life Chiropractic College West, she practiced chiropractic for a year in San Jose, Costa Rica, before returning to the Bay Area to open her current chiropractic practice. She just added "mother" to her resume and lives with her husband and daughter in the San Francisco Bay Area.

Anna V. Zulaica is a certified holistic nutrition consultant who has been working in the food and beverage industry for over 12 years. She has worked in Silicon Valley's corporate culinary setting, both as a cook and as a food and beverage program manager. Anna founded and ran Presto! Catering and Food Services, where she taught workshops and courses on healthy cooking for over five years, and currently teaches healthy cooking classes and workshops for the American Heart Association in Spanish and English throughout the Bay Area. Anna's recipes have been published in *The Antioxidant Counter: A Pocket Guide to the Revolutionary ORAC Scale for Choosing Healthy Foods* and she has coauthored two books, *The DASH Diet Cookbook: Quick and Delicious Recipes for Losing Weight, Preventing Diabetes, and Lowering Blood Pressure* and *The Low GI Slow Cooker: Delicious and Easy Dishes Made Healthy with the Glycemic Index.*

Lasheeda Perry spends her early mornings creating sweet (but not too sweet) scratch-made pastries and desserts as the executive pastry chef for a Silicon Valley company. Originally from the City of Brotherly Love, Lasheeda has spent the past nine years studying and traveling the world since graduating in 2008 with a bachelor of science from Johnson & Wales University. She was a valued member of the Four Seasons Hotels and Resorts culinary team, sharing her pastry skills in Dallas, Philadelphia, Baltimore, Lanai, and most recently, Palo Alto.